KIDNEY STONE

COOKBOOK AND FOOD LIST

Nutritional Guide with a meal plan for
preventing kidney stones and recipes to
improve renal function

Dr. VICTORIA H. MILLER

1

Table of Contents

Chapter 1

Introduction

Understanding Kidney Stones

Kidney stones, scientifically known as renal calculi, are solid crystalline structures that form in the kidneys. These formations can vary widely in size and composition, ranging from small, sand-like particles to larger, more complex structures. While the exact cause of kidney stones can vary, they often develop when certain substances in the urine, such as calcium, oxalate, and phosphorus, become highly concentrated and precipitate into solid crystals.

Understanding the types of kidney stones, including calcium oxalate, struvite, uric acid, and cystine stones, is crucial for effective management. Dehydration, dietary factors, and genetic predisposition contribute to their formation, emphasizing the importance of lifestyle and dietary adjustments for prevention.

This introduction sets the stage for a deeper exploration into the causes, risk factors, and dietary considerations that play a significant role in kidney stone development. By gaining insights into these aspects, individuals can proactively adopt measures to reduce the risk of kidney stones and promote overall kidney health.

Types of Kidney Stones

Understanding the specific type of kidney stone is crucial for developing targeted prevention and treatment strategies. Diagnosis often involves analyzing a passed stone or using imaging techniques to identify the stone's composition. Tailoring interventions based on the type of stone helps in implementing dietary modifications, lifestyle changes, and medical treatments to reduce the risk of recurrence and manage symptoms effectively.

Below are types of kidney stone

1. **Calcium Oxalate Stones:**

• *Composition:* These stones are primarily composed of calcium and oxalate.

• *Formation:* Develop when there is an excess of calcium and oxalate in the urine, leading to the crystallization of these substances.

• *Contributing Factors:* High intake of oxalate-rich foods, inadequate fluid consumption, and certain medical conditions can contribute to the formation of calcium oxalate stones.

2. **Struvite Stones:**

• *Composition:* Comprised of magnesium, ammonium, and phosphate.

• *Formation:* Often associated with urinary tract infections, as bacteria produce urease, an enzyme that increases the alkalinity of the urine, promoting struvite crystal formation.

• *Contributing Factors:* Chronic urinary tract infections and conditions that promote alkaline urine.

3. **Uric Acid Stones:**

• *Composition:* Mainly consist of uric acid, a byproduct of the breakdown of purines.

• *Formation:* Develop when urine is persistently acidic, leading to the crystallization of uric acid.

- *Contributing Factors:* High intake of purine-rich foods (such as organ meats and certain seafood), dehydration, and conditions that increase uric acid production.

4. **Cystine Stones:**

- *Composition:* Composed of the amino acid cystine.

- *Formation:* Result from a genetic disorder called cystinuria, where the kidneys excrete excessive amounts of cystine, leading to its accumulation in the urinary tract.

- *Contributing Factors:* Genetic predisposition, as cystinuria is an inherited condition.

Causes and Risk Factors

Understanding these causes and risk factors is crucial for identifying individuals at risk and implementing preventative measures. Lifestyle modifications, dietary adjustments, and proper hydration are key components of kidney stone prevention strategies tailored to individual risk profiles.

Below are the causes and risk factor

1. **Dehydration:**

- *Cause:* Insufficient fluid intake leads to concentrated urine, increasing the likelihood of crystallized substances forming kidney stones.

- *Risk Factor:* Individuals who do not maintain proper hydration levels are at an increased risk of developing kidney stones.

2. **Dietary Factors:**

- *Cause:* Consumption of foods high in oxalates, calcium, and purines can contribute to the formation of specific types of kidney stones.

- *Risk Factor:* Diets rich in oxalate-containing foods (such as spinach and nuts), excessive calcium intake, and high-purine diets can elevate the risk of kidney stone development.

3. **Genetic Predisposition:**

- *Cause:* Inherited conditions, such as cystinuria, can lead to an overproduction of specific substances (e.g., cystine) that contribute to stone formation.

- *Risk Factor:* Individuals with a family history of kidney stones may have a genetic predisposition, increasing their susceptibility to stone development.

4. **Medical Conditions:**

- *Cause:* Certain medical conditions, including urinary tract infections, inflammatory bowel disease, and renal tubular acidosis, can create an environment conducive to stone formation.

- *Risk Factor:* Individuals with these conditions may have an elevated risk of kidney stones.

5. **Obesity:**

- *Cause:* Obesity is associated with various metabolic changes that can increase the risk of kidney stone formation.

- *Risk Factor:* Overweight individuals may have higher levels of urinary excretion of calcium and oxalate, contributing to stone development.

6. **Age and Gender:**

- *Cause:* The risk of kidney stones tends to increase with age.

- *Risk Factor:* Men are more likely than women to develop kidney stones, with the risk peaking in the 30-60 age range.

7. **Geographic Location:**

- *Cause:* The prevalence of kidney stones varies based on geographical factors, including climate and diet.

- *Risk Factor:* Regions with higher temperatures and lower humidity may see an increased incidence of kidney stones due to dehydration.

8. **Urinary Tract Anomalies:**

- *Cause:* Structural abnormalities in the urinary tract, such as blockages or narrow passages, can impede the normal flow of urine.

- *Risk Factor:* Individuals with congenital or acquired urinary tract anomalies may be at a higher risk of developing kidney stones.

Importance of Diet in Kidney Stone Prevention

Maintaining a well-balanced and kidney stone-friendly diet plays a crucial role in preventing the formation of kidney stones. Dietary choices influence the concentration of various substances in urine, affecting the likelihood of crystal formation.

Here's why diet is of paramount importance in kidney stone prevention:

1. **Hydration and Dilution:**

- *Importance:* Adequate fluid intake, primarily water, helps dilute the concentration of minerals and substances in the urine, reducing the risk of crystallization.

- *Action:* Staying well-hydrated ensures a higher urine volume, preventing the saturation of minerals that can lead to stone formation.

2. **Oxalate Regulation:**

- *Importance:* Certain types of kidney stones, such as calcium oxalate stones, are influenced by high dietary oxalate intake.

- *Action:* Managing the consumption of oxalate-rich foods, such as spinach, beets, and nuts, helps control oxalate levels in the urine.

3. **Calcium Balance:**

- *Importance:* Adequate calcium intake is essential for overall health, but an imbalance can contribute to stone formation.

- *Action:* Balancing calcium intake through dietary sources, such as dairy products, and avoiding excessive calcium supplementation helps prevent the formation of calcium-based stones.

4. **Reducing Sodium Intake:**

- *Importance:* High sodium intake can increase calcium excretion in the urine, contributing to stone formation.

- *Action:* Moderating sodium intake, avoiding highly processed foods, and adopting a low-sodium diet can help manage calcium levels in the urine.

5. **Limiting Animal Proteins:**

- *Importance:* Diets rich in animal proteins can increase the excretion of certain substances, such as uric acid, promoting stone formation.

- *Action:* Limiting the intake of red meat, poultry, and fish can help reduce the risk of uric acid and other types of stones.

6. **Maintaining a Healthy Weight:**

- *Importance:* Obesity is associated with metabolic changes that can increase the risk of kidney stone formation.

- *Action:* Adopting a balanced diet and engaging in regular physical activity contribute to weight management, reducing the risk of stone development.

7. **Monitoring Oxidative Stress:**

- *Importance:* Oxidative stress may play a role in kidney stone formation.

- *Action:* Consuming antioxidant-rich foods, such as fruits and vegetables, may help counteract oxidative stress and promote kidney health.

8. **Individualized Dietary Plans:**

- *Importance:* Each individual may have unique dietary needs and responses.

- *Action:* Working with healthcare professionals, including dietitians, to create personalized dietary plans based on specific stone composition and risk factors enhances the effectiveness of preventive measures.

Chapter 2

Kidney Stone-Friendly Foods

Water and Hydration: The Role of Adequate Hydration

1. **Temperature Regulation:** Sweating is the body's natural way of cooling down. Proper hydration helps regulate body temperature by enabling effective sweating during physical activity or exposure to heat.

2. **Nutrient Transport:** Water is a key component in the transportation of nutrients throughout the body. It helps carry essential nutrients to cells and facilitates the absorption of these nutrients in the digestive system.

3. **Joint Lubrication:** Hydration plays a role in maintaining the lubrication of joints.

Dehydration can lead to joint stiffness and discomfort.

4. **Detoxification:** Water is essential for the elimination of waste products and toxins from the body through urine and feces. It supports the proper functioning of the kidneys and liver.

5. **Cognitive Function:** Dehydration can impair cognitive function, affecting concentration, alertness, and overall mental performance. Staying hydrated is crucial for maintaining optimal brain function.

6. **Skin Health:** Proper hydration contributes to skin elasticity and helps prevent dryness. Dehydrated skin is more prone to wrinkles and other signs of aging.

24

Hydrating Foods and Infusions

Hydrating Foods:

1. **Fruits:** Many fruits have high water content, making them excellent hydrating snacks. Examples include watermelon, oranges, berries, and grapefruit.

2. **Vegetables:** Vegetables like cucumber, celery, lettuce, and zucchini are rich in water and can contribute to overall hydration.

3. **Soups and Broths:** Consuming soups and broths, especially those with a high water content, can be an effective way to stay hydrated while also obtaining essential nutrients.

4. **Yogurt:** Yogurt and other dairy products contain water and contribute to hydration. Additionally, they provide

25

essential nutrients like calcium and probiotics.

5. **Smoothies:** Blending fruits and vegetables into smoothies can be a tasty way to increase water intake. Adding yogurt or milk can further enhance hydration.

Hydrating Infusions:

1. **Herbal Teas:** Herbal teas, such as peppermint or chamomile, can be hydrating without the diuretic effects of caffeinated beverages. They are also often rich in antioxidants.

2. **Infused Water:** Adding natural flavors to water with ingredients like cucumber, mint, lemon, or berries can make it more enticing and enjoyable, encouraging increased water intake.

3. **Coconut Water:** Coconut water is a natural electrolyte-rich beverage that can help replenish fluids and minerals lost during physical activity.

4. **Aloe Vera Juice:** Aloe vera juice, when consumed in moderation, can contribute to hydration and may offer additional health benefits.

5. **Vegetable Juices:** Freshly squeezed vegetable juices, such as celery or cucumber juice, can be hydrating and provide essential vitamins and minerals.

Low-Oxalate Foods

Low-Oxalate Vegetables:

1. **Leafy Greens:**

   - Iceberg Lettuce

   - Romaine Lettuce

- Red Leaf Lettuce

- Boston Lettuce

2. **Cruciferous Vegetables:**

    - Broccoli (steamed or boiled)

    - Cauliflower

    - Cabbage (green and red)

    - Bok Choy

3. **Root Vegetables:**

    - Carrots

    - Sweet Potatoes

    - Radishes

4. **Bell Peppers:**

    - Green Bell Peppers

    - Red Bell Peppers

    - Yellow Bell Peppers

5. **Zucchini and Summer Squash**

6. **Onions and Garlic:**

   - Yellow Onions

   - White Onions

   - Garlic

7. **Mushrooms:**

   - Button Mushrooms

   - Cremini Mushrooms

   - Portobello Mushrooms

8. **Asparagus**

9. **Green Beans**

10. **Cucumbers**

Low-Oxalate Fruits:

1. **Melons:**

    - Watermelon

    - Cantaloupe

    - Honeydew

2. **Berries:**

    - Strawberries

    - Blueberries

    - Raspberries

    - Blackberries

3. **Grapes:**

    - Red Grapes

    - Green Grapes

4. **Peaches**

5. **Nectarines**

6. **Pineapple**

7. **Cherries**

8. **Plums**

9. **Apples:**

   - Red Apples

   - Green Apples

10. **Pears:**

- Bartlett Pears

- Anjou Pears

Calcium-Rich Options

Calcium is an essential mineral that plays a crucial role in maintaining bone health, nerve function, and blood clotting. While dairy products are often rich in calcium, there are also non-dairy sources for individuals who may be lactose intolerant, follow a vegan diet, or choose not to consume dairy for other reasons.

Here's a list of both dairy and non-dairy sources of calcium:

Dairy Sources:

Milk:

- Cow's Milk (whole, reduced-fat, or skim)
- Goat's Milk

Cheese:

- Cheddar
- Mozzarella
- Swiss
- Parmesan

Yogurt:

- Greek Yogurt
- Regular Yogurt

Buttermilk

Cottage Cheese

Kefir

Ice Cream and Frozen Yogurt

Non-Dairy Sources:

Leafy Greens:

- Kale
- Collard Greens
- Turnip Greens
- Bok Choy
- Broccoli (especially if consumed in larger quantities)

Fortified Plant Milks:

- Almond Milk (fortified)
- Soy Milk (fortified)
- Rice Milk (fortified)
- Oat Milk (fortified)

Fortified Juices:

- Orange Juice (fortified with calcium)

- Other fruit juices (fortified)

Tofu and Tempeh:

- Firm Tofu
- Tempeh

Nuts and Seeds:

- Almonds
- Chia Seeds
- Sesame Seeds

Fish:

- Canned Fish with Bones (such as sardines and salmon)

Beans and Legumes:

- Chickpeas (Garbanzo Beans)
- White Beans
- Black Beans

Certain Vegetables:

- Okra

- Sweet Potatoes
- Acorn Squash

Fig Paste

Amaranth and Quinoa

Chapter 3

Lifestyle Strategies for Kidney Stone Prevention

Physical Activity and Kidney Health

Exercise Recommendations:

1.   Cardiovascular Exercise:

Aim for at least 150 minutes of moderate-intensity aerobic exercise per week or 75 minutes of vigorous-intensity aerobic exercise. Examples include brisk walking, jogging, cycling, or swimming.

2.   Strength Training:

Include strength training exercises at least two days a week. This can involve lifting weights, using resistance bands, or practicing bodyweight exercises like push-ups and squats.

3. **Flexibility Exercises:**

Incorporate flexibility exercises, such as stretching or yoga, into your routine. This can help improve overall mobility and reduce the risk of muscle strain.

4. **Stay Active Throughout the Day:**

Avoid prolonged periods of sitting or sedentary behavior. Take short breaks to stand, stretch, or walk, especially if you have a desk job.

5. **Hydrate Before and After Exercise:**

Drink plenty of water before, during, and after exercise to stay well-hydrated. Proper hydration can help prevent the formation of certain types of kidney stones.

Lifestyle Recommendations:

Maintain a Healthy Weight:

Aim for a healthy body weight through a combination of regular exercise and a balanced diet. Obesity is a risk factor for kidney stones.

Dietary Modifications:

Follow a diet rich in fruits, vegetables, and whole grains. Limit sodium, animal proteins, and foods high in oxalates, such as beets, chocolate, tea, and nuts. Consult with a healthcare professional or a registered dietitian for personalized dietary advice.

Limit Caffeine and Alcohol:

Excessive caffeine and alcohol intake can contribute to dehydration, which may increase the risk of kidney stone formation. Moderation is key.

Monitor Calcium Intake:

Ensure an adequate but not excessive intake of calcium. While calcium is essential for bone health, excessive intake from supplements may increase the risk of certain types of kidney stones.

Manage Stress:

Chronic stress can contribute to various health issues, including kidney stone formation. Incorporate stress-reducing activities such as meditation, deep breathing, or hobbies into your routine.

Regular Health Check-ups:

Schedule regular check-ups with your healthcare provider. They can monitor your overall health, assess kidney function, and provide guidance on kidney stone prevention.

Stress Management: The Impact of Stress on Kidney Health

1. **Blood Pressure Elevation:**

Chronic stress can lead to an increase in blood pressure, which is a risk factor for kidney disease. Elevated blood pressure can damage the blood vessels in the kidneys, affecting their ability to filter and regulate fluids.

2. **Hormonal Changes:**

Stress activates the body's "fight or flight" response, releasing stress hormones such as cortisol and adrenaline. Prolonged exposure to these hormones can affect the kidneys and contribute to imbalances in fluid and electrolyte regulation.

3.   **Behavioral Changes:**

Individuals experiencing stress may adopt unhealthy coping mechanisms, such as poor dietary choices, inadequate hydration, and a sedentary lifestyle. These behaviors can contribute to the formation of kidney stones.

4.   **Impact on Immune Function:**

Chronic stress may weaken the immune system, making the body more susceptible to infections. Kidney infections, if left untreated, can lead to complications affecting kidney function.

Relaxation Techniques for Kidney Stone Prevention

Meditation:

Mindfulness meditation and other meditation techniques can help reduce stress and promote relaxation. Taking a few minutes each day to focus on your breath and quiet your mind can be beneficial.

Deep Breathing Exercises:

Practice deep breathing exercises to activate the body's relaxation response. Slow, deep breaths can help calm the nervous system and reduce stress.

Progressive Muscle Relaxation (PMR):

PMR involves tensing and then gradually releasing different muscle groups, promoting physical and mental relaxation. This technique can be helpful in reducing overall tension.

Yoga:

Yoga combines physical postures, breath control, and meditation. Regular practice can promote relaxation, improve flexibility, and reduce stress.

Tai Chi:

Tai Chi is a gentle martial art that involves slow, flowing movements and deep breathing. It has been shown to reduce stress and improve overall well-being.

Guided Imagery:

Visualization and guided imagery involve creating mental images that promote relaxation. This technique can be used to create a sense of calm and reduce stress.

Aromatherapy:

Certain scents, such as lavender or chamomile, are known for their calming effects. Using essential oils or aromatherapy can create a soothing environment.

Massage Therapy:

Massage can help relax muscles, reduce tension, and alleviate stress. Regular massages may contribute to overall well-being.

Chapter 4

Kidney Stone-Friendly Food List

A kidney stone-friendly diet aims to reduce the risk of kidney stone formation by managing the intake of certain minerals and compounds that can contribute to stone development. The most common types of kidney stones are calcium oxalate stones, uric acid stones, and struvite stones.

Here's a kidney stone-friendly food list, taking into consideration various dietary factors:

Low-Oxalate Foods:

Leafy Greens:

- Iceberg Lettuce
- Romaine Lettuce
- Red Leaf Lettuce
- Kale (in moderation)
- Spinach (in moderation)

Cruciferous Vegetables:

- Broccoli (cooked)
- Cauliflower
- Brussels Sprouts
- Bok Choy

Root Vegetables:

- Carrots
- Sweet Potatoes

Bell Peppers:

- Green Bell Peppers
- Red Bell Peppers
- Yellow Bell Peppers

Zucchini and Summer Squash

Onions and Garlic:

- Yellow Onions
- White Onions
- Garlic

Fruits:

- Melons (watermelon, cantaloupe)
- Berries (strawberries, blueberries, raspberries)
- Apples
- Grapes

Pears:

- Bartlett Pears
- Anjou Pears

Cucumbers

Dairy:

- Low-fat or fat-free Milk
- Yogurt
- Cheese (in moderation)

Low-Purine Foods (for Uric Acid Stones):

Lean Proteins:

- Chicken
- Turkey
- Fish (salmon, trout)
- Eggs

Dairy:

- Low-fat or fat-free Milk
- Yogurt
- Cheese (in moderation)

Plant-Based Proteins:

- Tofu
- Lentils
- Chickpeas

Fruits:

- Cherries
- Berries

Low-Sodium Foods:

Fresh Fruits and Vegetables

Lean Proteins:

- Chicken
- Turkey
- Fish

Whole Grains:

- Quinoa
- Brown Rice

Nuts and Seeds (in moderation):

- Almonds
- Walnuts
- Chia Seeds
- Flaxseeds

Hydrating Foods:

Water-Rich Fruits:

- Watermelon

- Cucumber
- Berries

Soups and Broths (low-sodium):

- Vegetable Soup
- Chicken Broth

Foods to Limit or Avoid:

High-Oxalate Foods:

- Beets
- Chocolate
- Tea
- Nuts

High-Purine Foods (for Uric Acid Stones):

- Red Meat
- Organ Meats (liver, kidneys)
- Shellfish

High-Sodium Foods:

- Processed Foods

- Canned Soups
- Fast Food

Excessive Animal Proteins:

Reducing excessive intake of meat, eggs, and dairy, especially in those prone to forming calcium oxalate stones.

Chapter 5

28 day Meal Plan for Kidney Stone Prevention

Week 1

Day 1:

Breakfast: Greek yogurt parfait with mixed berries and a sprinkle of chia seeds

Lunch: Quinoa salad with chickpeas, cherry tomatoes, cucumbers, and a lemon-tahini dressing

Dinner: Grilled chicken breast with steamed broccoli and quinoa

Snack: Sliced apple with a tablespoon of almond butter

Day 2:

Breakfast: Oatmeal with sliced peaches and a dollop of Greek yogurt

Lunch: Lentil soup with whole-grain crackers

Dinner: Baked salmon with asparagus and wild rice

Snack: Carrot and cucumber sticks with hummus

Day 3:

Breakfast: Spinach and feta omelet with whole-grain toast

Lunch: Turkey and avocado wrap with a side of carrot sticks

Dinner: Stir-fried tofu with bok choy, bell peppers, and brown rice

Snack: Greek yogurt with a handful of walnuts

Day 4:

Breakfast: Smoothie with kale, banana, almond milk, and a scoop of protein powder

Lunch: Caprese salad with fresh mozzarella, tomatoes, and basil

Dinner: Shrimp and vegetable stir-fry with quinoa

Snack: Fresh berries with a sprinkle of sunflower seeds

Day 5:

Breakfast: Whole-grain waffles with strawberries and a dollop of Greek yogurt

Lunch: Chickpea and vegetable curry with brown rice

Dinner: Grilled tilapia with lemon-dill sauce, sweet potato wedges, and green beans

Snack: Cottage cheese with pineapple chunks

Day 6:

Breakfast: Scrambled eggs with spinach, tomatoes, and whole-grain toast

Lunch: Mediterranean salad with mixed greens, olives, feta cheese, and a light vinaigrette

Dinner: Baked chicken breast with quinoa pilaf and sautéed zucchini

Snack: Handful of unsalted almonds

Day 7:

Breakfast: Avocado and tomato on whole-grain toast

Lunch: Black bean and corn salad with avocado and cilantro

Dinner: Grilled steak (moderate portion) with roasted sweet potatoes and broccoli

Snack: Popcorn (air-popped) with a sprinkle of nutritional yeast

Week 2

Day 8:

Breakfast: Smoothie with spinach, banana, almond milk, and a scoop of protein powder

Lunch: Quinoa and black bean bowl with salsa, avocado, and cilantro

Dinner: Baked cod with lemon-dill sauce, sweet potato mash, and green beans

Snack: Fresh berries with a dollop of Greek yogurt

Day 9:

Breakfast: Greek yogurt parfait with mixed berries and a sprinkle of granola

Lunch: Turkey and vegetable stir-fry with brown rice

Dinner: Grilled chicken Caesar salad with romaine lettuce and cherry tomatoes

Snack: Handful of unsalted pistachios

Day 10:

Breakfast: Scrambled eggs with tomatoes and whole-grain toast

Lunch: Chickpea and spinach curry with quinoa

Dinner: Grilled shrimp with quinoa pilaf and roasted vegetables

Snack: Cottage cheese with pineapple chunks

Day 11:

Breakfast: Whole-grain pancakes with sliced peaches and a drizzle of honey

Lunch: Lentil and vegetable soup with a side of whole-grain crackers

Dinner: Baked chicken thighs with rosemary, sweet potato wedges, and asparagus

Snack: Carrot and cucumber sticks with hummus

Day 12:

Breakfast: Oatmeal with mixed berries and a spoonful of almond butter

Lunch: Quinoa salad with cherry tomatoes, cucumber, and feta cheese

Dinner: Grilled salmon with a quinoa and black bean salad

Snack: Fresh fruit salad with a squeeze of lime

Day 13:

Breakfast: Smoothie with kale, pineapple, coconut water, and a scoop of protein powder

Lunch: Turkey and avocado wrap with a side of carrot sticks

Dinner: Stir-fried tofu with broccoli, bell peppers, and brown rice

Snack: Greek yogurt with a handful of walnuts

Day 14:

Breakfast: Avocado toast on whole-grain bread

Lunch: Caprese salad with fresh mozzarella, tomatoes, and basil

Dinner: Baked cod with lemon-butter sauce, quinoa, and green beans

Snack: Popcorn (air-popped) with a sprinkle of nutritional yeast

Week 3

Day 15:

Breakfast: Greek yogurt with mixed berries and a sprinkle of granola

Lunch: Quinoa and black bean bowl with salsa, avocado, and cilantro

Dinner: Grilled chicken Caesar salad with romaine lettuce and cherry tomatoes

Snack: Handful of unsalted pistachios

Day 16:

Breakfast: Scrambled eggs with tomatoes and whole-grain toast

Lunch: Chickpea and spinach curry with quinoa

Dinner: Grilled shrimp with quinoa pilaf and roasted vegetables

Snack: Cottage cheese with pineapple chunks

Day 17:

Breakfast: Whole-grain pancakes with sliced peaches and a drizzle of honey

Lunch: Lentil and vegetable soup with a side of whole-grain crackers

Dinner: Baked chicken thighs with rosemary, sweet potato wedges, and asparagus

Snack: Carrot and cucumber sticks with hummus

Day 18:

Breakfast: Oatmeal with mixed berries and a spoonful of almond butter

Lunch: Quinoa salad with cherry tomatoes, cucumber, and feta cheese

Dinner: Grilled salmon with a quinoa and black bean salad

Snack: Fresh fruit salad with a squeeze of lime

Day 19:

Breakfast: Smoothie with kale, pineapple, coconut water, and a scoop of protein powder

Lunch: Turkey and avocado wrap with a side of carrot sticks

Dinner: Stir-fried tofu with broccoli, bell peppers, and brown rice

Snack: Greek yogurt with a handful of walnuts

Day 20:

Breakfast: Avocado toast on whole-grain bread

Lunch: Caprese salad with fresh mozzarella, tomatoes, and basil

Dinner: Baked cod with lemon-butter sauce, quinoa, and green beans

Snack: Popcorn (air-popped) with a sprinkle of nutritional yeast

Day 21:

Breakfast: Greek yogurt with mixed berries and a sprinkle of granola

Lunch: Quinoa and black bean bowl with salsa, avocado, and cilantro

Dinner: Grilled chicken Caesar salad with romaine lettuce and cherry tomatoes

Snack: Handful of unsalted pistachios

Week 4

Day 22:

Breakfast: Scrambled eggs with tomatoes and whole-grain toast

Lunch: Chickpea and spinach curry with quinoa

Dinner: Grilled shrimp with quinoa pilaf and roasted vegetables

Snack: Cottage cheese with pineapple chunks

Day 23:

Breakfast: Whole-grain pancakes with sliced peaches and a drizzle of honey

Lunch: Lentil and vegetable soup with a side of whole-grain crackers

Dinner: Baked chicken thighs with rosemary, sweet potato wedges, and asparagus

Snack: Carrot and cucumber sticks with hummus

Day 24:

Breakfast: Oatmeal with mixed berries and a spoonful of almond butter

Lunch: Quinoa salad with cherry tomatoes, cucumber, and feta cheese

Dinner: Grilled salmon with a quinoa and black bean salad

Snack: Fresh fruit salad with a squeeze of lime

Day 25:

Breakfast: Smoothie with kale, pineapple, coconut water, and a scoop of protein powder

Lunch: Turkey and avocado wrap with a side of carrot sticks

Dinner: Stir-fried tofu with broccoli, bell peppers, and brown rice

Snack: Greek yogurt with a handful of walnuts

Day 26:

Breakfast: Avocado toast on whole-grain bread

Lunch: Caprese salad with fresh mozzarella, tomatoes, and basil

Dinner: Baked cod with lemon-butter sauce, quinoa, and green beans

Snack: Popcorn (air-popped) with a sprinkle of nutritional yeast

Day 27:

Breakfast: Greek yogurt with mixed berries and a sprinkle of chia seeds

Lunch: Quinoa and black bean bowl with salsa, avocado, and cilantro

Dinner: Grilled chicken Caesar salad with romaine lettuce and cherry tomatoes

Snack: Handful of unsalted pistachios

Day 28:

Breakfast: Scrambled eggs with tomatoes and whole-grain toast

Lunch: Chickpea and spinach curry with quinoa

Dinner: Grilled shrimp with quinoa pilaf and roasted vegetables

Snack: Cottage cheese with pineapple chunks

Chapter 6

Breakfast Recipes for Kidney Stone Prevention

Greek Yogurt Parfait:

Ingredients:

- 1 cup Greek yogurt

- 1/2 cup mixed berries (blueberries, strawberries, raspberries)

- 2 tablespoons granola

- 1 tablespoon chia seeds

Instructions:

1. In a glass or bowl, layer Greek yogurt.

2. Add a layer of mixed berries.

3. Sprinkle granola and chia seeds on top.

4. Repeat layers as desired.

Nutritional Information:

- Calories: 300

- Protein: 20g

- Carbohydrates: 30g

- Fat: 12g

- Fiber: 6g

Vegetable Omelet:

Ingredients:

- 2 eggs

- 1/4 cup bell peppers, diced

- 1/4 cup tomatoes, diced

- 2 tablespoons feta cheese

- 1 teaspoon olive oil

Instructions:

1. Whisk eggs in a bowl.

2. Heat olive oil in a pan and sauté bell peppers and tomatoes.

3. Pour whisked eggs over vegetables.

4. Sprinkle feta cheese on top and cook until eggs are set.

Nutritional Information:

- Calories: 250

- Protein: 18g

- Carbohydrates: 7g

- Fat: 17g

- Fiber: 2g

Oatmeal with Fresh Fruit:

Ingredients:

- 1/2 cup rolled oats
- 1 cup almond milk
- 1/2 banana, sliced

- 1/4 cup berries
- 1 tablespoon almond butter

Instructions:

1. Cook oats in almond milk until creamy.
2. Top with sliced banana, berries, and a dollop of almond butter.

Nutritional Information:

- Calories: 320
- Protein: 9g
- Carbohydrates: 46g
- Fat: 12g
- Fiber: 8g

Whole-Grain Waffles with Berries:

Ingredients:

- 2 whole-grain waffles
- 1/2 cup mixed berries
- 2 tablespoons Greek yogurt
- 1 tablespoon honey

Instructions:

1. Toast whole-grain waffles.

2. Top with mixed berries, Greek yogurt, and a drizzle of honey.

Nutritional Information:

- Calories: 280

- Protein: 8g

- Carbohydrates: 50g

- Fat: 5g

- Fiber: 6g

Avocado Toast:

Ingredients:
- 2 slices whole-grain bread
- 1/2 avocado, mashed
- Cherry tomatoes, sliced
- Sprinkle of black pepper

Instructions:

1. Toast whole-grain bread slices.

2. Spread mashed avocado on the toast.

3. Top with sliced cherry tomatoes and black pepper.

Nutritional Information:

- Calories: 230

- Protein: 6g

- Carbohydrates: 25g

- Fat: 13g

- Fiber: 8g

Smoothie Bowl:

Ingredients:

- 1 cup spinach

- 1/2 banana

- 1/2 cup pineapple chunks

- 1/2 cup almond milk

- Toppings: Chia seeds, sliced strawberries, and granola

Instructions:

1. Blend spinach, banana, pineapple, and almond milk until smooth.

2. Pour into a bowl and top with chia seeds, sliced strawberries, and granola.

Nutritional Information:

- Calories: 280

- Protein: 7g

- Carbohydrates: 54g

- Fat: 6g

- Fiber: 10g

Quinoa Breakfast Bowl:

Ingredients:

- 1/2 cup cooked quinoa

- 1/4 cup sliced almonds

- 1/2 cup mixed berries

- 1 tablespoon honey

Instructions:

1. Combine cooked quinoa, sliced almonds, and mixed berries in a bowl.

2. Drizzle with honey.

Nutritional Information:

- Calories: 280

- Protein: 8g

- Carbohydrates: 45g

- Fat: 8g

- Fiber: 6g

Chia Seed Pudding:

Ingredients:

- 2 tablespoons chia seeds
- 1 cup almond milk
- 1/2 teaspoon vanilla extract
- 1/2 cup mango chunks

Instructions:

1. Mix chia seeds, almond milk, and vanilla extract in a jar. Refrigerate overnight.
2. Top with mango chunks before serving.

Nutritional Information:

- Calories: 210
- Protein: 5g
- Carbohydrates: 30g
- Fat: 9g

- Fiber: 11g

Whole-Grain Pancakes with Berries:

Ingredients:

- 2 whole-grain pancakes

- 1/2 cup mixed berries

- 2 tablespoons Greek yogurt

- 1 tablespoon maple syrup

Instructions:

1. Cook whole-grain pancakes according to package instructions.

2. Top with mixed berries, Greek yogurt, and a drizzle of maple syrup.

Nutritional Information:

- Calories: 320

- Protein: 10g

- Carbohydrates: 60g

- Fat: 5g

- Fiber: 8g

Egg and Vegetable Breakfast Wrap:

Ingredients:

- 1 whole-grain wrap

- 2 eggs, scrambled

- 1/4 cup bell peppers, diced

- 1/4 cup black beans, cooked

- Salsa for topping

Instructions:

1. Cook scrambled eggs with diced bell peppers and black beans.

2. Fill a whole-grain wrap with the egg mixture.

3. Top with salsa.

Nutritional Information:

- Calories: 320

- Protein: 20g

- Carbohydrates: 35g

- Fat: 12g

- Fiber: 8g

Chapter 7

Lunchtime Favourite for Kidney Stone Prevention

Grilled Chicken Salad:

Ingredients:

- 4 oz grilled chicken breast, sliced

- Mixed greens (lettuce, spinach)

- Cherry tomatoes, halved

- Cucumber, sliced

- 1 tablespoon olive oil

- Balsamic vinegar for dressing

Instructions:

1. Arrange mixed greens on a plate.

2. Top with grilled chicken, cherry tomatoes, and cucumber.

3. Drizzle with olive oil and balsamic vinegar.

Nutritional Information:

- Calories: 350

- Protein: 30g

- Carbohydrates: 10g

- Fat: 20g

- Fiber: 4g

Quinoa and Black Bean Bowl:

Ingredients:

- 1/2 cup cooked quinoa

- 1/2 cup black beans, cooked

- 1/4 cup corn kernels

- 1/4 cup diced bell peppers

- Salsa for topping

Instructions:

1. Mix cooked quinoa, black beans, corn, and bell peppers in a bowl.

2. Top with salsa before serving.

Nutritional Information:

- Calories: 300

- Protein: 12g

- Carbohydrates: 55g

- Fat: 3g

- Fiber: 10g

Mediterranean Chickpea Salad:

Ingredients:

- 1 cup chickpeas, drained and rinsed

- Cucumber, diced

- Cherry tomatoes, halved

- Red onion, finely chopped

- Feta cheese, crumbled

- Olive oil and lemon juice for dressing

Instructions:

1. Combine chickpeas, cucumber, tomatoes, red onion, and feta in a bowl.

2. Dress with olive oil and lemon juice.

Nutritional Information:

- Calories: 280

- Protein: 11g

- Carbohydrates: 40g

- Fat: 10g

- Fiber: 9g

Turkey and Avocado Wrap:

Ingredients:

- 4 oz turkey breast slices
- Whole-grain wrap
- Avocado, sliced
- Lettuce leaves
- Mustard for flavor

Instructions:

1. Lay out the whole-grain wrap.
2. Add turkey, avocado slices, lettuce, and mustard.
3. Roll up and enjoy.

Nutritional Information:

- Calories: 320
- Protein: 25g

- Carbohydrates: 30g

- Fat: 12g

- Fiber: 8g

Vegetarian Quinoa Stir-Fry:

Ingredients:

- 1/2 cup cooked quinoa

- Mixed vegetables (broccoli, bell peppers, carrots)

- Tofu, cubed

- Soy sauce for seasoning

- Sesame oil for stir-frying

Instructions:

1. Stir-fry mixed vegetables and tofu in sesame oil.

2. Add cooked quinoa and soy sauce.

3. Toss until well combined.

Nutritional Information:

- Calories: 280

- Protein: 15g

- Carbohydrates: 40g

- Fat: 10g

- Fiber: 8g

Salmon and Quinoa Salad:

Ingredients:

- 4 oz baked or grilled salmon

- 1/2 cup cooked quinoa

- Mixed greens

- Cherry tomatoes, halved

- Cucumber, sliced

- Lemon-tahini dressing

Instructions:

1. Arrange mixed greens on a plate.

2. Top with baked or grilled salmon, quinoa, tomatoes, and cucumber.

3. Drizzle with lemon-tahini dressing.

Nutritional Information:

- Calories: 380

- Protein: 30g

- Carbohydrates: 20g

- Fat: 20g

- Fiber: 4g

Lentil and Vegetable Soup:

Ingredients:

- 1 cup cooked lentils

- Mixed vegetables (carrots, celery, onions)

- Low-sodium vegetable broth

- Garlic and herbs for flavor

Instructions:

1. Sauté mixed vegetables in a pot with garlic.

2. Add cooked lentils and vegetable broth.

3. Season with herbs and simmer until vegetables are tender.

Nutritional Information:

- Calories: 250

- Protein: 15g

- Carbohydrates: 40g

- Fat: 2g

- Fiber: 10g

Caprese Salad with Grilled Chicken:

Ingredients:

- 4 oz grilled chicken breast, sliced

- Tomatoes, sliced

- Fresh mozzarella, sliced

- Fresh basil leaves

- Balsamic glaze for drizzling

Instructions:

1. Arrange sliced tomatoes, mozzarella, and grilled chicken on a plate.

2. Top with fresh basil leaves.

3. Drizzle with balsamic glaze.

Nutritional Information:

- Calories: 320

- Protein: 30g

- Carbohydrates: 10g

- Fat: 18g

- Fiber: 2g

Chickpea and Spinach Curry:

Ingredients:

- 1 cup chickpeas, drained and rinsed

- Fresh spinach leaves

- Coconut milk

- Curry spices (turmeric, cumin, coriander)

- Brown rice for serving

Instructions:

1. Simmer chickpeas, spinach, and coconut milk in curry spices.

2. Serve over brown rice.

Nutritional Information:

- Calories: 320

- Protein: 15g

- Carbohydrates: 50g

- Fat: 10g

- Fiber: 12g

Baked Cod with Lemon-Dill Sauce:

Ingredients:

- 6 oz cod fillet

- Lemon juice

- Fresh dill, chopped

- Olive oil

- Quinoa or steamed vegetables for serving

Instructions:

1. Place cod on a baking sheet.

2. Drizzle with lemon juice, olive oil, and sprinkle with chopped dill.

3. Bake until fish is cooked through. Serve with quinoa or steamed vegetables.

Nutritional Information:

- Calories: 250

- Protein: 30g

- Carbohydrates: 10g

- Fat: 10g

- Fiber: 2g

Chapter 8

Dinner Delicacy for Kidney Stone Prevention

Grilled Salmon with Lemon-Dill Sauce:

Ingredients:

- 6 oz salmon fillet
- Lemon juice
- Fresh dill, chopped
- Olive oil
- Steamed broccoli and quinoa for serving

Instructions:

1. Grill salmon, drizzle with lemon juice, and sprinkle with chopped dill.

2. Serve over steamed broccoli and quinoa.

Nutritional Information:

- Calories: 350

- Protein: 30g

- Carbohydrates: 20g

- Fat: 15g

- Fiber: 5g

Stir-Fried Tofu with Vegetables:

Ingredients:

- Firm tofu, cubed

- Mixed vegetables (bell peppers, broccoli, snap peas)

- Soy sauce

- Ginger and garlic for flavor

- Brown rice for serving

Instructions:

1. Stir-fry tofu and mixed vegetables in soy sauce, ginger, and garlic.

2. Serve over brown rice.

Nutritional Information:

- Calories: 320

- Protein: 15g

- Carbohydrates: 45g

- Fat: 12g

- Fiber: 8g

Baked Chicken Breast with Quinoa Pilaf:

Ingredients:

- 6 oz chicken breast

- Lemon zest and juice

- Fresh parsley, chopped

- Quinoa pilaf (quinoa, diced vegetables, olive oil)

Instructions:

1. Season chicken with lemon zest and juice, bake until cooked.

2. Serve with quinoa pilaf topped with fresh parsley.

Nutritional Information:

- Calories: 300

- Protein: 35g

- Carbohydrates: 25g

- Fat: 8g

- Fiber: 5g

Vegetarian Chickpea and Spinach Curry:

Ingredients:

- Chickpeas, drained and rinsed

- Fresh spinach leaves

- Coconut milk

- Curry spices (turmeric, cumin, coriander)

- Brown rice for serving

Instructions:

1. Simmer chickpeas, spinach, and coconut milk in curry spices.

2. Serve over brown rice.

Nutritional Information:

- Calories: 320

- Protein: 15g

- Carbohydrates: 50g

- Fat: 10g

- Fiber: 12g

Grilled Turkey Burgers with Sweet Potato Wedges:

Ingredients:

- Turkey burger patties

- Whole-grain burger buns

- Sweet potato wedges, baked

- Lettuce, tomato, and onion for topping

Instructions:

1. Grill turkey burger patties.

2. Serve in whole-grain buns with baked sweet potato wedges.

Nutritional Information:

- Calories: 380

- Protein: 25g

- Carbohydrates: 40g

- Fat: 15g

- Fiber: 8g

Lentil and Vegetable Stir-Fry:

Ingredients:

- Cooked lentils
- Mixed vegetables (bell peppers, carrots, broccoli)
- Soy sauce
- Garlic and ginger for flavor
- Brown rice for serving

Instructions:

1. Stir-fry cooked lentils and mixed vegetables in soy sauce, garlic, and ginger.
2. Serve over brown rice.

Nutritional Information:

- Calories: 300

- Protein: 18g

- Carbohydrates: 50g

- Fat: 4g

- Fiber: 10g

Baked Cod with Tomato and Olive Relish:

Ingredients:

- 6 oz cod fillet

- Tomatoes, diced

- Kalamata olives, sliced

- Fresh basil, chopped

- Olive oil for drizzling

Instructions:

1. Place cod on a baking sheet.

2. Top with diced tomatoes, olives, and fresh basil.

3. Drizzle with olive oil and bake until fish is cooked through.

Nutritional Information:

- Calories: 280
- Protein: 30g
- Carbohydrates: 10g
- Fat: 15g
- Fiber: 3g

Chickpea and Quinoa Stuffed Bell Peppers:

Ingredients:

- Bell peppers, halved
- Cooked quinoa
- Chickpeas, mashed
- Diced tomatoes and onions
- Italian herbs for seasoning

Instructions:

1. Mix cooked quinoa, mashed chickpeas, diced tomatoes, onions, and Italian herbs.

2. Stuff bell peppers and bake until peppers are tender.

Nutritional Information:

- Calories: 320

- Protein: 15g

- Carbohydrates: 50g

- Fat: 8g

- Fiber: 10g

Shrimp Stir-Fry with Brown Rice:

Ingredients:

- Shrimp, peeled and deveined

- Mixed vegetables (broccoli, bell peppers, snap peas)
- Soy sauce
- Ginger and garlic for flavor
- Brown rice for serving

Instructions:

1. Stir-fry shrimp and mixed vegetables in soy sauce, ginger, and garlic.
2. Serve over brown rice.

Nutritional Information:

- Calories: 340
- Protein: 25g
- Carbohydrates: 45g
- Fat: 6g
- Fiber: 8g

Eggplant and Tomato Casserole:

Ingredients:

- Eggplant, sliced

- Tomatoes, sliced

- Mozzarella cheese, shredded

- Fresh basil leaves

- Olive oil for drizzling

Instructions:

1. Layer sliced eggplant and tomatoes in a baking dish.

2. Top with shredded mozzarella and fresh basil.

3. Drizzle with olive oil and bake until bubbly.

Nutritional Information:

- Calories: 280

- Protein: 12g

- Carbohydrates: 20g

- Fat: 18g

- Fiber: 8g

Chapter 9

Snacks and Treats for Kidney Stone Prevention

Greek Yogurt and Berry Parfait:

Ingredients:

- 1 cup Greek yogurt
- 1/2 cup mixed berries (blueberries, strawberries, raspberries)
- 2 tablespoons granola
- 1 tablespoon honey

Instructions:

1. In a glass or bowl, layer Greek yogurt.
2. Add a layer of mixed berries.
3. Sprinkle granola on top and drizzle with honey.

Nutritional Information:

- Calories: 250
- Protein: 15g

- Carbohydrates: 35g

- Fat: 8g

- Fiber: 4g

Cottage Cheese and Pineapple Cups:

Ingredients:

- 1 cup low-fat cottage cheese

- 1/2 cup fresh pineapple chunks

- Mint leaves for garnish

Instructions:

1. Divide cottage cheese into serving cups.

2. Top with fresh pineapple chunks.

3. Garnish with mint leaves.

Nutritional Information:

- Calories: 200

- Protein: 20g

- Carbohydrates: 25g

- Fat: 2g

- Fiber: 2g

Homemade Trail Mix:

Ingredients:

- Almonds, walnuts, and pistachios

- Dried apricots and cranberries

- Dark chocolate chips

Instructions:

1. Mix together desired amounts of nuts, dried fruits, and dark chocolate chips.

2. Portion into small snack bags for easy grabbing.

Nutritional Information:

- Calories: 180

- Protein: 5g

- Carbohydrates: 20g

- Fat: 10g

- Fiber: 4g

Vegetable Sticks with Hummus:

Ingredients:

- Carrot and cucumber sticks
- Hummus for dipping

Instructions:

1. Cut carrots and cucumbers into sticks.
2. Serve with a side of hummus for dipping.

Nutritional Information:

- Calories: 120
- Protein: 4g
- Carbohydrates: 15g
- Fat: 6g
- Fiber: 6g

Popcorn with Nutritional Yeast:

Ingredients:

- Air-popped popcorn

- Nutritional yeast

Instructions:

1. Pop popcorn using an air popper.

2. Sprinkle nutritional yeast over the popcorn for a savory flavor.

Nutritional Information:

- Calories: 80

- Protein: 3g

- Carbohydrates: 15g

- Fat: 1g

- Fiber: 3g

Apple Slices with Almond Butter:

Ingredients:

- Apple slices
- Almond butter

Instructions:

1. Slice apples into wedges.
2. Spread almond butter on each slice.

Nutritional Information:

- Calories: 150
- Protein: 3g
- Carbohydrates: 20g
- Fat: 8g
- Fiber: 5g

Smoothie Bowl with Nut Butter:

Ingredients:

- 1 cup mixed berries (frozen or fresh)
- 1/2 banana

- 1/2 cup almond milk

- Toppings: Sliced almonds, chia seeds, and a spoonful of nut butter

Instructions:

1. Blend berries, banana, and almond milk until smooth.

2. Pour into a bowl and top with sliced almonds, chia seeds, and a spoonful of nut butter.

Nutritional Information:

- Calories: 300

- Protein: 10g

- Carbohydrates: 40g

- Fat: 15g

- Fiber: 8g

Chia Seed Pudding with Fresh Fruit:

Ingredients:

- 2 tablespoons chia seeds

- 1 cup almond milk

- 1/2 teaspoon vanilla extract

- Fresh berries for topping

Instructions:

1. Mix chia seeds, almond milk, and vanilla extract in a jar. Refrigerate overnight.

2. Top with fresh berries before serving.

Nutritional Information:

- Calories: 200

- Protein: 5g

- Carbohydrates: 30g

- Fat: 9g

- Fiber: 11g

Roasted Chickpeas:

Ingredients:

- 1 can chickpeas, drained and rinsed
- Olive oil
- Smoked paprika and cumin for seasoning

Instructions:

1. Toss chickpeas with olive oil and seasonings.
2. Roast in the oven until crispy.

Nutritional Information:

- Calories: 160
- Protein: 6g
- Carbohydrates: 25g
- Fat: 5g
- Fiber: 7g

Frozen Banana Pops:

Ingredients:

- Bananas, peeled and halved
- Greek yogurt
- Dark chocolate, melted
- Chopped nuts for coating

Instructions:

1. Dip banana halves in Greek yogurt and freeze.
2. Once frozen, dip in melted dark chocolate and coat with chopped nuts.

Nutritional Information:

- Calories: 180
- Protein: 5g
- Carbohydrates: 30g
- Fat: 8g

- Fiber: 4g

Chapter 10

Conclusion

In conclusion, the Kidney Stone Cookbook and Food List not only serves as a comprehensive guide to delicious and nutritious recipes but also empowers individuals to take proactive steps towards kidney stone prevention through mindful dietary choices. By incorporating a wide array of low-oxalate, kidney-friendly foods and hydrating infusions, this cookbook provides a versatile culinary approach that is both satisfying and supportive of optimal kidney health.

The incorporation of low-oxalate vegetables and fruits, along with the right sources of calcium from both dairy and non-dairy options, forms a balanced foundation for meals that prioritize kidney stone prevention. Furthermore, the inclusion of exercise and stress-management strategies underscores the holistic approach to overall well-being, acknowledging the interconnectedness of lifestyle factors in kidney health.

Understanding the impact of stress on kidney health and the role of relaxation techniques not only adds depth to this culinary guide but emphasizes the importance of a harmonious mind-body relationship in preventing kidney stones. By recognizing the potential stressors and offering effective relaxation methods, this cookbook extends beyond a mere collection of recipes, fostering a holistic approach to kidney stone prevention that considers both dietary and lifestyle factors.

The meticulously crafted 28-day meal plan, inclusive of snacks and treats, is a practical and user-friendly tool for individuals seeking to make lasting dietary changes. From nutrient-packed breakfasts to wholesome dinners and satisfying snacks, the meal plan ensures variety and flavor while adhering to kidney stone prevention principles. Each day is thoughtfully designed, catering to diverse tastes and preferences, thereby making the journey towards optimal kidney health an enjoyable and sustainable one.

Ultimately, the Kidney Stone Cookbook and Food List not only equips individuals with the knowledge and tools to make kidney-friendly choices but also instills a sense of empowerment and control over one's own health. As we savor the delicious recipes and embrace a kidney stone-friendly lifestyle, we embark on a journey towards improved well-being, with the cookbook serving as a trusted companion on the path to lasting kidney health.

Printed in Great Britain
by Amazon

46256182R00066